SOMATIC EXERCISES FOR WEIGHT LOSS

By Smith J. Offor

Table of Contents

Introduction

Somatic exercise is a fascinating practice that focuses on the mind-body connection and encourages us to move with awareness and intention. Somatic exercise involves a series of movements and exercises designed to increase body awareness, release tension, and improve overall movement patterns. Let's explore this practice further and discover its benefits and key principles.

Mindful Movement

Somatic exercise emphasizes mindful movement, where you bring conscious awareness to the sensations in your body as you engage in different exercises. It's about being fully present and attentive to how your body moves, allowing you to develop a deeper connection with your physical self.

Body Sensing

Somatic exercise encourages body sensing, which involves tuning in to the subtle sensations and messages your body sends. By cultivating body awareness, you can detect areas of tension, imbalances, or restricted movement. This heightened awareness enables you to address these issues and promote greater freedom of movement.

Neuromuscular Re-Education

Somatic exercise aims to re-educate the neuromuscular system, which includes the muscles, nerves, and brain. Through specific movements and exercises, you can release habitual patterns of tension and reprogram your body to move with greater efficiency, ease, and fluidity.

Slow and Gentle Practice

Somatic exercise is typically slow and gentle, allowing you to explore movements in a controlled and deliberate manner. By moving slowly, you can engage with the sensory feedback from your body more effectively, bringing attention to the details of each movement.

Pandiculation

Pandiculation is a key principle of somatic exercise. It involves a three-step process of contracting, releasing, and lengthening muscles to reset their resting length. By pandiculating, you can release chronic muscular tension

and restore optimal muscle
function.

Proprioception and Kinesthetic Awareness

Somatic exercise enhances
proprioception, which is your
body's ability to perceive its
position and movement in space.
It also improves kinesthetic
awareness, which is your sense of
body position and motion.
Developing these skills through
somatic exercise helps you move
with greater precision, balance,
and coordination.

Whole-Body Integration

Somatic exercise views the body
as a whole, interconnected system.
Instead of isolating individual
muscles or body parts, it focuses
on integrating movements and
engaging multiple muscle groups

simultaneously. This approach promotes functional movement patterns and overall body balance.

Breath and Relaxation
Just like in somatic yoga, somatic exercise emphasizes the importance of breath and relaxation. Deep, diaphragmatic breathing helps promote relaxation, release tension, and support the mind-body connection. By incorporating breath awareness into your somatic exercise practice, you can enhance its benefits.

Incorporating somatic exercise into your fitness routine can be a transformative experience. It allows you to develop a deeper understanding of your body, release tension, and improve movement patterns. Whether you're a beginner or an experienced fitness enthusiast, somatic exercise offers a unique approach to exercise that can enhance your overall well-being.

What are the types of somatic exercises?

Let's explore the wonderful world of somatic exercises and the different types you can engage in to enhance your mind-body connection and overall well-being. Somatic exercises encompass a wide range of movements and techniques that promote body awareness, release tension, and improve movement patterns. Here are a few types of somatic exercises you can explore:

Somatic Movement Exercises

Somatic movement exercises involve slow, mindful, and intentional movements that focus on reprogramming the neuromuscular system. These exercises often incorporate pandiculation, which is the contraction, release, and lengthening of muscles to reset their resting length. Somatic movement exercises can help release chronic muscular tension, improve flexibility, and enhance body awareness.

Somatic Yoga

Somatic yoga combines the principles of somatic movement with traditional yoga poses and sequences. It emphasizes mindful movement, breath awareness, and the release of tension in the body. Somatic yoga can help improve flexibility, balance, and relaxation while promoting a deeper connection with your body.

Feldenkrais Method

The Feldenkrais Method is a somatic education system that focuses on improving movement patterns and body awareness. It consists of gentle movements, both done actively and passively, to explore new possibilities of movement and release habitual patterns of tension. The Feldenkrais Method can be practiced through group classes or individual sessions called Functional Integration.

Alexander Technique

The Alexander Technique is a somatic practice that focuses on improving posture, movement, and overall body coordination. It involves learning to release unnecessary muscular tension, aligning the body in a balanced manner, and moving with ease and efficiency. The Alexander Technique is often taught through individual lessons with a certified teacher.

Body-Mind Centering

Body-Mind Centering is a somatic practice that integrates movement, touch, and visualization to explore the interconnectedness of the body and mind. It involves embodying different body systems, such as organs, bones, and fluids, to deepen body awareness and enhance movement potential.

Body-Mind Centering can be experienced through classes, workshops, or individual sessions.

Hanna Somatics

Hanna Somatics, developed by Thomas Hanna, focuses on releasing chronic muscular tension and improving movement patterns through a series of gentle and slow exercises. It involves a combination of pandiculation, mindful movement, and self-awareness to bring about lasting changes in the body. Hanna Somatics exercises can be practiced independently or with the guidance of a certified practitioner.

Remember, these are just a few examples of somatic exercises, and there are many more approaches and variations within the somatic field. Exploring different types of somatic exercises allows you to find what resonates with you and supports your unique journey towards greater body awareness, release of tension, and improved movement patterns.

What are the benefits of somatic exercise?

The benefits of somatic exercise are truly remarkable! Engaging in this practice can have a profound impact on your overall well-being, both physically and mentally. Let's delve into some of the key benefits of somatic exercise:

Improved Body Awareness

Somatic exercise helps you

develop a deeper connection with your body and enhances your body awareness. By paying close attention to the sensations, movements, and messages your body sends, you become more attuned to its needs and can address any imbalances or areas of tension.

Release of Tension and Stress
Somatic exercise is an effective tool for releasing chronic muscular tension and reducing stress levels. The slow, deliberate movements and mindful approach enable you to identify areas of tension and consciously release them, promoting relaxation and a sense of ease in the body.

Enhanced Movement Patterns

Engaging in somatic exercise can improve your movement patterns and overall physical function. By re-educating the neuromuscular system, you can release habitual patterns of movement that may be causing restrictions or discomfort. This, in turn, allows for greater freedom, efficiency, and fluidity of movement.

Increased Flexibility and Range of Motion

Somatic exercise can help improve flexibility and increase your range of motion. By releasing tension and addressing muscular imbalances, you can experience greater ease and suppleness in your movements. This can be particularly beneficial for individuals who experience stiffness or limited mobility.

Better Posture and Alignment

Somatic exercise focuses on improving postural alignment and body mechanics. By cultivating awareness of your posture and engaging in movements that promote proper alignment, you can reduce postural imbalances, alleviate strain on the body, and support optimal postural function.

Stress Reduction and Relaxation

Somatic exercise offers an opportunity for stress reduction and relaxation. The slow, intentional movements, combined with breath awareness and mindfulness, help activate the relaxation response in the body. This can help reduce stress levels, promote a sense of calm, and improve overall well-being.

Mind-Body Connection

Somatic exercise enhances the mind-body connection, allowing you to develop a deeper understanding of how your thoughts, emotions, and physical sensations interrelate. By bringing awareness to the present moment and fostering a connection with your body, you can cultivate a greater sense of overall balance and harmony.

Improved Emotional Well-being

Engaging in somatic exercise can have a positive impact on your emotional well-being. By releasing tension and promoting relaxation, you can experience a reduction in anxiety and stress levels.

Additionally, the mind-body connection fostered through somatic exercise can help cultivate a greater sense of self-awareness and emotional resilience.

Rehabilitation and Injury Prevention

Somatic exercise can be beneficial for rehabilitation and injury prevention. By addressing imbalances, releasing tension, and improving movement patterns, somatic exercise can support the healing process and reduce the risk of future injuries. It can also be a valuable complement to other rehabilitation modalities.

Overall Mind-Body Integration

Ultimately, somatic exercise promotes overall mind-body integration. By incorporating movement, breath awareness, and mindfulness, you can cultivate a holistic approach to well-being that encompasses both the physical and mental aspects of your being.

The benefits of somatic exercise are vast and multifaceted, offering a comprehensive approach to enhancing your overall well-being. By embracing this practice, you can experience improved body awareness, reduced tension and stress, enhanced movement patterns, and a deeper connection with your mind and body.

Somatic exercises for weight loss: Do they work?

The quest for weight loss, a topic that many of us are curious about. When it comes to somatic exercises specifically targeting weight loss, it's important to understand their role and how they can contribute to your overall weight loss journey. Let's explore!

Somatic exercises may not be the primary focus for weight loss, as they are more geared towards improving body awareness, releasing tension, and enhancing movement patterns. However, they can still play a valuable role in your weight loss efforts. Here's how:

Mindful Eating

Somatic exercises promote mindfulness and body awareness, which can extend to your eating habits. By being more in tune with your body and its signals, you can develop a greater awareness of hunger and fullness cues. This can help prevent overeating and support healthier eating patterns, ultimately contributing to weight management.

Stress Reduction

Somatic exercises can be effective in reducing stress levels, which is crucial for weight management. Stress often triggers emotional eating or cravings for unhealthy foods. By incorporating somatic exercises into your routine, you can help reduce stress and manage emotional eating, leading to better weight control.

19

Improved Body Composition

While somatic exercises may not
directly burn a significant number
of calories, they can improve your
body composition. By releasing
tension and improving movement
patterns, somatic exercises help
optimize muscle function and
alignment. This can result in
better muscle tone, posture, and
overall body shape, even if the
number on the scale doesn't
change drastically.

Movement Variety

Adding somatic exercises to your
fitness routine can provide variety
and prevent exercise plateau. By
engaging in different types of
movements, you challenge your
body in new ways, which can boost
metabolism and calorie burning.
This, in turn, can support weight
loss efforts when combined with a

well-rounded exercise program
and a balanced diet.

Enhanced Overall Well-being
Somatic exercises promote overall
well-being, including mental and
emotional health. When you feel
good mentally and emotionally,
you are more likely to make
positive choices for your body,
including maintaining a healthy
weight. Somatic exercises can
contribute to a positive mindset,
self-care, and a holistic approach
to weight management.

While somatic exercises alone may
not lead to significant weight loss,
incorporating them into a
comprehensive weight loss plan
can be beneficial. It's important to
combine somatic exercises with
other forms of exercise, such as
cardiovascular activities and

strength training, as well as adopt a balanced and nutritious diet. Remember, sustainable weight loss is a result of a combination of lifestyle factors, including exercise, nutrition, sleep, and stress management.

Do somatic exercises help with belly fat?

While somatic exercises may not directly target belly fat specifically, they can still contribute to overall weight management and body composition, which includes reducing excess fat in the abdominal area. Let's explore how somatic exercises can play a role in addressing belly fat:

Improved Posture

Somatic exercises focus on improving postural alignment and body mechanics. By addressing postural imbalances and promoting proper alignment, somatic exercises can help lengthen and strengthen the core muscles, including the muscles in the abdominal area. This can lead to improved posture and a more toned appearance in the abdominal region.

Enhanced Core Strength

Somatic exercises often incorporate movements that engage the core muscles. These exercises can help strengthen the deep abdominal muscles, such as the transverse abdominis and the obliques. Strengthening these muscles can provide stability and support to the spine, improve core strength, and contribute to a flatter and more toned belly.

Increased Muscle Tone: Somatic exercises promote neuromuscular re-education, which helps release tension and improve movement patterns. By engaging in somatic exercises, you can enhance muscle tone throughout the body, including the abdominal muscles. While these exercises may not directly burn belly fat, they can contribute to a more sculpted and toned midsection.

Stress Reduction

Somatic exercises are effective in reducing stress levels, and stress can contribute to the accumulation of belly fat. By incorporating somatic exercises into your routine, you can help manage stress and reduce the production of cortisol, a hormone associated with increased abdominal fat storage. Stress reduction can indirectly support belly fat reduction efforts.

Overall Weight Management
Somatic exercises, when combined with a balanced diet and other forms of exercise, can contribute to overall weight management. While spot reduction (targeting fat loss in specific areas) is not possible, engaging in regular physical activity, including somatic exercises, can help create a calorie deficit, which is essential for losing excess body fat, including belly fat.

It's important to note that reducing belly fat requires a comprehensive approach that includes a balanced diet, regular exercise, and overall lifestyle modifications. Somatic exercises can be a valuable addition to this approach, but they are most effective when combined with other forms of exercise, such as cardiovascular activities and strength training, and a healthy, calorie-controlled diet.

FAQs

Can somatic exercises alone reduce belly fat?

Somatic exercises alone may not lead to significant belly fat reduction. Spot reduction of fat in specific areas is not possible through exercise alone. However, incorporating somatic exercises into a comprehensive weight management plan, which includes a balanced diet and other forms of exercise, can contribute to overall body fat reduction, including in the abdominal area.

How long does it take to see results in belly fat reduction with somatic exercises?

The timeline for seeing results in belly fat reduction can vary from person to person and depends on various factors, including genetics, overall body composition, diet, and exercise habits. It's important to approach belly fat reduction with patience and consistency. With regular practice of somatic exercises, combined with a healthy lifestyle, it is possible to see improvements in body composition over time.

Are there specific somatic exercises that target belly fat?
While somatic exercises may not specifically target belly fat, there are exercises that can engage the core muscles, including the abdominal muscles. Examples include gentle abdominal contractions, pelvic tilts, and mindful breathing exercises that activate the deep core muscles. Incorporating these exercises into your somatic practice can contribute to overall core strength and toning of the abdominal area.

Mindful Movement: Unlocking the Power of Somatic Exercises for Weight Loss

When it comes to achieving weight loss and overall wellness, exercise is a crucial component. However, many of us overlook the importance of mindful movement and somatic exercises in our journey towards a healthier body. In this article, we'll explore the role of somatic exercises in weight loss, focusing on how they can help reduce stress and promote a positive body image.

The Connection Between Stress and Weight Gain

Stress is a common phenomenon that can have a profound impact on our physical and emotional well-being. When we experience stress, our bodies release cortisol, a hormone that can increase appetite and lead to cravings for high-calorie comfort foods. Additionally, stress can disrupt our sleep patterns, influencing our hunger and satiety hormones and making it challenging to maintain a healthy weight.

Somatic Exercises: A Path to Reduced Stress and Improved Weight Loss

Somatic exercises focus on enhancing the mind-body connection through mindful movement. These targeted exercises aim to release tension from the body, promote relaxation, and optimize the functioning of the nervous system. By engaging in somatic exercises, we can activate the parasympathetic nervous system, which is responsible for the body's "rest and digest" response. This not only reduces stress but also sets the stage for effective weight loss.

Beyond Physical Benefits: Cultivating Introspection and Body Awareness

Unlike traditional workout routines that focus primarily on burning calories, somatic exercises offer more than just physical benefits. They provide a pathway to explore the underlying causes of stress and weight issues, allowing us to cultivate introspection and body awareness. By incorporating somatic exercises into our daily routine, we can develop a deeper understanding of our body's needs and address the root causes of stress and emotional eating.

The Power of Mindset in Weight Management

While mindset plays a significant role in weight management, it's essential to recognize that physical sensations are also crucial for achieving success. By bridging the gap between mind and body through somatic exercises, we can tap into our body's natural wisdom and unlock transformative weight loss results.

Cultivating a Positive Body Image Through Nervous System Regulation

Somatic exercises play a crucial role in regulating the nervous system, which can bring about incredible benefits such as enhanced mood, sustained energy levels, and a greater sense of peace and freedom in the body. By actively participating in nervous system regulation through somatic exercises, we can boost self-esteem and develop a more positive body image.

Incorporating Somatic Exercises into Your Weight Loss Plan

If you're considering incorporating somatic exercises into your weight loss plan, it's essential to find what works best for you. You can start with simple exercises like yoga or tai chi, or try using an app like NEUROFIT that offers a range of somatic exercises to support your

weight loss journey. Remember,
even just a few minutes each day
can make a significant difference.

3 Somatic Exercises to Support Your Weight Loss Goals

The Cannon: Up-regulate Your Nervous System

Stand up, inhale, and stretch your arms out wide to the side. Retain your breath while slowly squeezing your arms in, as if closing a heavy door. Exhale powerfully through your mouth and release.

ENS Massage: Increase Interoception

Gently massage your stomach in round motions, beginning at the belly button and moving outwards. Concentrate on how you feel and the beat.

Wall Presses: Down-Regulate Your Nervous System

Press steadily against a wall for a few seconds, then release and repeat. Exhale as you push and inhale as you release.

Somatic exercises offer a holistic approach to weight loss by addressing the underlying factors that contribute to weight gain. By incorporating mindful movement and somatic release techniques into your daily routine, you can reduce stress, regulate your nervous system, and develop a more positive body image. Remember, weight loss is not just about diet and exercise; it's about understanding and addressing the root causes of stress and emotional eating. By embracing somatic exercises and cultivating a healthy mindset, you can unlock transformative weight loss results.

Slow Burn: A Somatic Approach to Exercise

I recently had the pleasure of reading "Slow Burn," an exceptional book by Stu Mittleman, an accomplished ultra-distance-running champion. Stu holds the US record for running 578 miles in just 6 days, which amounts to an astounding 96 miles per day! While I initially picked up the book hoping to learn how to maximize fat burn during workouts (which I did, and I'll share those insights later), what truly captivated me was Stu's unique somatic approach to training. This approach is a rarity in the fitness world but can be applied to any type of exercise that you enjoy.

"Slow Burn" is an inspirational read that I believe should be on the list of every athlete and non-athlete alike. For athletes, it will challenge your perspectives on warm-ups, training methods, body connection, and fueling for optimal performance. And if you're not an athlete, this book will give you the confidence and knowledge you need to start exercising at a slow pace while staying connected to your body, avoiding injuries, shedding weight, and improving strength and endurance.

Stu's Somatic Approach to Exercise

Back in 1983, Stu embarked on his first six-day race without proper preparation. He had never run for more than 24 hours at a time. Stu's initial strategy was to run until he couldn't run anymore, then rest until he felt ready to run again. Unfortunately, this approach quickly led to burnout, and by the second day, he was ready to quit.

Thankfully, a fellow runner shared a life-changing revelation with Stu. The top runners had a structured schedule: they ran for a predetermined time and then rested for a predetermined period. They repeated this pattern, never allowing themselves to become depleted. They rested before reaching exhaustion, which enabled them to stay in control and maintain productivity throughout the race.

Stu immediately adopted this approach and created a repeatable schedule that worked for him. At the end of the six days, he finished the race in second place, setting a new American record.

Taking the Path of Least Resistance

This experience led Stu to develop a somatic approach to exercise. Instead of focusing solely on pace, he shifted his attention to the experience of running itself. Stu's priority became how effectively he could manage his state, rather than how fast he could run.

Stu beautifully explains, "Life is a marathon, not a sprint, and you must prepare accordingly. Unlike sprinters who focus on reaching the finish line as fast as possible, endurance athletes have no finish line. They must remain connected to their bodies, in tune with every move, in a place that feels comfortable and productive, and

that they can maintain
indefinitely."

In the book, Stu emphasizes the
importance of developing a
relationship with your body to
successfully navigate through a
marathon, whether it's a literal
race or the marathon of life. Treat
your body as your partner, listen
to its messages, and avoid forcing
it to do things it doesn't want to
do. Instead, work with your body,
taking the path of least resistance
rather than subscribing to the "no
pain, no gain" mentality.

Partnering with Your Body
By paying attention to your body's
signals, you become the expert in
your own health. Stu emphasizes

that no health professional can make better decisions about your well-being than you. It's crucial to acquire knowledge from experts and become as informed as possible. Combine that knowledge with a highly attuned sense of your body's needs to make the best decisions for your health.

Another key aspect of Stu's training approach aligns perfectly with somatics: focusing on the process rather than fixating solely on the end goal. This shift in mindset can be challenging at first, especially for those new to somatic exercises. Slowing down and immersing yourself in the sensations of movement, rather than counting repetitions or anticipating the finish line, is a

transformative experience.
Somatic exercises allow for
gradual change to occur, leading to
profound shifts in the body.

Process-Oriented Goals: A Somatic Approach to Exercise

Applying this approach to fitness training presents its own set of challenges. How can you get faster or stronger without setting specific goals? Stu suggests setting "process-oriented goals" that focus on maintaining awareness of your breathing, form, comfort level, and heart rate. This advice significantly impacted my own exercise routine. Previously, I approached my runs with the mindset that faster was always better, constantly pushing myself to the limit. Negative self-talk would flood my mind, questioning why I wasn't faster or in better shape.

Applying Stu's approach, I experienced immediate results. By slowing down my pace and prioritizing my breathing and heart rate, I effortlessly increased my distance, burned more calories, and found greater enjoyment in my runs. The pressure to achieve specific goals disappeared, allowing me to relax and fully embrace the experience. Stu Mittleman's somatic approach reminded me that exercise isn't just about achieving an end result; it's about the journey and the connection with our bodies.

The Mind-Body Connection

Stu's somatic approach highlights the crucial mind-body connection in exercise. It's not just about the physical exertion; it's about being present in the moment and fully engaging with your body's sensations. By focusing on the experience rather than the outcome, you can cultivate a deeper connection with your body and enhance your overall well-being.

Mindful Movement and Injury Prevention

One of the key benefits of adopting a somatic approach to exercise is injury prevention. When we rush through our workouts or push ourselves too hard, we increase the risk of injury. By practicing mindful movement and listening to our bodies, we can avoid overexertion and give ourselves the necessary rest and recovery.

Building Strength from Within

Stu's approach also emphasizes building strength from within. It's not just about the external appearance or pushing our limits; it's about developing resilience and inner strength. By focusing on the process and nurturing our bodies, we can cultivate a sustainable and long-lasting fitness journey.

Integrating Somatic Exercises
While Stu's book primarily focuses on running, his somatic approach can be applied to any form of exercise. Whether it's yoga, weightlifting, swimming, or dancing, the principles of mindful movement, body awareness, and listening to your body's cues are universal.

"Slow Burn" by Stu Mittleman is a remarkable book that challenges the traditional notions of exercise and introduces a somatic approach to fitness training. By prioritizing the mind-body connection, focusing on the process rather than the outcome, and listening to our bodies, we can create a sustainable and fulfilling exercise routine. Remember, it's not just about the destination; it's about

the journey and the connection
with our bodies.

FAQs

1. How can I apply the somatic approach to my exercise routine?

To apply the somatic approach to
your exercise routine, start by
prioritizing the mind-body
connection. Focus on being
present in the moment, fully
engaging with your body's
sensations, and listening to its
cues. Slow down and pay attention
to your breathing, form, comfort
level, and heart rate. Set process-
oriented goals that emphasize the

experience rather than specific outcomes. By doing so, you can cultivate a deeper connection with your body and enhance your overall well-being.

2. Can the somatic approach help prevent injuries during exercise?

Yes, adopting a somatic approach to exercise can help prevent injuries. By practicing mindful movement, listening to your body, and avoiding overexertion, you can reduce the risk of strains, sprains, and other exercise-related injuries. The somatic approach encourages you to give your body the rest and recovery it needs, ultimately promoting a safer and more sustainable exercise routine.

3. Is the somatic approach limited to specific types of exercise?

No, the somatic approach can be applied to any form of exercise. Whether you prefer yoga, weightlifting, swimming, or dancing, the principles of mindful movement, body awareness, and listening to your body's cues are universal. The somatic approach is about developing a deeper connection with your body and prioritizing its needs, regardless of the specific type of exercise you engage in.

Stored Trauma in Your Body: The Hidden Culprit Behind Weight Gain and Inability to Lose It

Have you ever felt stuck in your weight loss journey, despite putting in consistent effort at the gym and maintaining a healthy diet? If so, you're not alone. Many people struggle to shed those stubborn pounds, and the answer might lie in something deeper than just exercise and nutrition. It could be stored trauma in your body.

Meet Liz Tenuto, also known as 'The Workout Witch' on Instagram and YouTube. Liz has amassed a devoted following by advocating for a compassionate approach to fitness. She believes that incorporating somatic exercises and stress relief techniques into your routine can help you address the stored trauma that might be hindering your weight loss progress.

Understanding the Impact of Trauma on Weight Gain

Trauma can manifest in various forms, such as emotional, physical, or psychological distress. When we experience trauma, our bodies often go into survival mode, triggering a stress response. This response can lead to a release of stress hormones like cortisol, which can impact our metabolism and contribute to weight gain.

The Link Between Trauma and Weight Loss Resistance

Even with a dedicated fitness regimen and a well-balanced diet, some individuals struggle to lose weight. This resistance could be attributed to unaddressed trauma. Liz emphasizes the importance of delving deeper into the root causes of weight gain and exploring somatic exercises as a means to release stored trauma.

What Are Somatic Exercises?

Somatic exercises involve gentle movements and mindfulness techniques that aim to reconnect your mind and body. These exercises promote body awareness, release tension, and allow you to tap into the innate wisdom of your body. By engaging in somatic exercises, you can address the emotional and physical aspects of trauma, laying the foundation for sustainable weight loss.

The Benefits of Somatic Exercises for Weight Loss

Stress Reduction: Somatic exercises help alleviate stress and promote relaxation, reducing the release of cortisol and allowing your body to function optimally.

Emotional Healing: By addressing stored trauma, somatic exercises can help you process emotions related to past experiences, fostering emotional well-being and reducing emotional eating.

Improved Body Awareness: Somatic exercises enhance your mind-body connection, enabling you to listen to your body's signals of hunger and satisfaction more effectively.

Enhanced Metabolism: Releasing tension and stress from your body through somatic exercises can support a healthy metabolism and improve your body's ability to burn calories.

Incorporating Somatic Exercises into Your Routine

If you're interested in exploring somatic exercises to release stored trauma and aid in weight loss, here are a few simple practices you can incorporate into your daily routine:

Body Scan Meditation: Take a few minutes each day to scan your body, noticing any areas of tension or discomfort. Slowly release the tension and breathe deeply, allowing your body to relax.

Yoga or Tai Chi: Engage in gentle movement practices like yoga or Tai Chi to promote body awareness, flexibility, and stress reduction.

Deep Breathing Exercises: Practice deep breathing exercises to calm your nervous system, reduce stress, and promote relaxation.

Mindful Eating: Pay attention to the sensations of eating, savoring each bite and listening to your body's cues of hunger and fullness.

Journaling: Write down your thoughts and feelings, allowing yourself to process emotions related to past traumas.

Remember, everyone's journey is unique, and it's essential to listen to your body and seek professional guidance if needed. Somatic exercises can be a powerful tool in your weight loss journey, helping you release stored trauma and create a healthier relationship with your body.

FAQs

Can trauma really contribute to weight gain?

Yes, trauma can trigger a stress response in the body, leading to the release of stress hormones like cortisol. This can impact metabolism and contribute to weight gain.

How can somatic exercises help with weight loss?

Somatic exercises promote body awareness, release tension, and address stored trauma. By engaging in these exercises, you can reduce stress, process emotions, and enhance your metabolism, ultimately supporting your weight loss journey.

Are somatic exercises suitable for everyone?

Somatic exercises can be beneficial for many individuals, but it's essential to listen to your body and consult with a healthcare professional if you have any underlying health conditions or concerns. They can provide personalized guidance based on your specific needs.

www.ingramcontent.com/pod-product-compliance
Lightning Source LLC
Chambersburg PA
CBHW051845250726
48659CB00006B/2040